Unveiling Submission

Embracing the Power of Surrender

Bella Horne

PROLOGUE: A GLIMPSE INTO THE UNVEILING

In the depths of the human psyche lies a tapestry of desires and yearnings, woven intricately with threads of power, control, and vulnerability. It is a realm often shrouded in mystery, misconceptions, and societal taboos. Yet, for those who dare to venture beyond the surface, a world of profound connection, self-discovery, and liberation awaits.

"Unveiling Submission: Embracing the Power of Surrender" invites you to embark on a journey of exploration, a journey that transcends boundaries and challenges preconceived notions. Here, within the pages that lie before you, we delve into the depths of submission—a path where power dynamics intertwine, where trust and consent dance, and where vulnerability becomes a source of empowerment.

In this world, submission is not synonymous with weakness, but rather a conscious choice—a surrender that reveals hidden strength and unspoken desires. It is a journey that extends far beyond the bedroom, permeating everyday life, relationships, and the essence of self.

Through the words and experiences shared within these pages, you will encounter the essence of submission—the core principles and motivations that drive individuals to embrace a submissive role. We will break down the misconceptions and stereotypes that often cloud our understanding, illuminating the beauty and authenticity that lies within the world of submission.

As we delve deeper, we will explore the foundation upon which submission is built—consent, trust, and effective communication. We will uncover the power of choice, the significance of boundaries, and the tools that ensure safety and well-being in submissive experiences. We will navigate the delicate balance between independence and surrender, where personal growth and empowerment flourish.

Rituals, protocols, and the intertwining of dominance and submission will be unveiled, shedding light on the intricacies of the dynamic. We will witness how power dynamics shape daily life, routines, and interactions, and how rewards, punishments, and discipline contribute to structure and accountability.

As we journey further, we will venture into the realm of desires and kinks, embracing the diversity and complexity of BDSM practices. We will explore the taboo, the edges of darkness, and the challenges of exploring those hidden corners while ensuring the safety and well-being of all involved.

Ultimately, this exploration of submission is not just about physical acts, but a transformative journey of self-discovery and personal growth. We will unravel the layers of the self, where vulnerability becomes a source of strength and surrender becomes an avenue for authenticity.

As you embark on this journey, let the words on these pages be your guide. Open your mind, shed the layers of societal constraints, and allow the power of submission to unfold before you. Embrace the essence of surrender, and may this unveiling ignite within you a newfound understanding, acceptance, and empowerment.

So, let us venture forth together, into the depths of submission, and unravel the tapestry of desires that lie within. Let us embark on a journey that transcends boundaries, challenges perceptions, and uncovers the power that lies within the embrace of surrender. Welcome to "Unveiling Submission: Embracing the Power of Surrender."

CHAPTER 1: THE ESSENCE OF SUBMISSION: EXPLORING THE CORE PRINCIPLES AND MOTIVATIONS BEHIND EMBRACING A SUBMISSIVE ROLE.

Exploring Core Principles and Motivations.

Submission is a multifaceted concept that goes beyond stereotypes and preconceived notions. It is a journey of self-discovery, trust, and profound connection. In this chapter, we will delve into the essence of submission, exploring its core principles and motivations that inspire individuals to embrace a submissive role.

Defining Submission: Submission, in its essence, is the act of willingly relinquishing power and control to another person, known as the dominant. It is a consensual exchange that creates a dynamic where one person takes the lead, while the other finds fulfilment in surrendering.

Trust and Safety: Central to submission is the foundation of trust. Trust is the bedrock upon which the submissive dynamic is built. The submissive places their well-being, emotional vulnerability, and physical safety in the hands of their dominant partner. Trust is earned over time through open communication, understanding, and the consistent demonstration of respect and care.

Desire for Surrender: The motivation to embrace submission stems from a deep-seated desire for surrender. Some individuals find fulfilment, freedom, and even empowerment in letting go of control and embracing vulnerability. The act of surrendering can provide a sense of relief from the pressures and responsibilities of daily life, allowing the submissive to find solace in the trust they place in their dominant.

Emotional Intimacy and Connection: Submission often fosters an unparalleled level of emotional intimacy and connection between the submissive and the dominant. The power dynamics involved in submission create a unique space for vulnerability and trust to flourish. Through their shared experiences, the dominant and submissive build a deep bond that extends beyond physical intimacy.

Personal Growth and Exploration: The journey of submission offers a path of personal growth and self-discovery. By embracing the submissive role, individuals often gain a deeper understanding of their own desires, boundaries, and strengths. The exploration of submission can challenge societal norms, foster self-acceptance, and enable personal empowerment.

Service and Fulfilment: For some submissives, the act of service plays a significant role in their motivation to embrace submission. Serving their dominant partner's needs, whether through acts of physical service, emotional support, or fulfilling specific tasks, brings a sense of purpose and fulfilment.

Freedom Within Boundaries: Contrary to misconceptions, submission is not synonymous with oppression or lack of agency. In a healthy submissive dynamic, boundaries are established and respected, creating a framework that allows the submissive to explore their desires within negotiated limits. Submission provides a unique freedom found in surrendering control to a trusted dominant partner.

The essence of submission lies in the principles of trust, surrender, emotional intimacy, personal growth, and service. It is a consensual exchange of power that allows individuals to explore their desires, embrace vulnerability, and foster deep connections. Understanding these core principles and motivations is crucial for those embarking on the journey of submission, as it sets the stage for a fulfilling and empowering experience.

CHAPTER 2: ADDRESSING COMMON MYTHS AND STEREOTYPES SURROUNDING SUBMISSION

Submission is often shrouded in misconceptions and stereotypes, perpetuated by society's limited understanding and portrayal of alternative relationships and dynamics. In this chapter, we will debunk common myths and stereotypes surrounding submission, shedding light on the reality and diversity of submissive experiences.

Myth 1: Submissives are Weak or Inferior: One prevalent misconception is that submissives are weak individuals who lack agency or self-confidence. In reality, submission requires immense strength, self-awareness, and the ability to trust and communicate effectively. Submissives actively choose to embrace their desires and willingly surrender control, demonstrating courage and resilience.

Myth 2: Dominants are Abusive or Controlling: A damaging stereotype is that dominants are inherently abusive or seek to exert control over their submissive partners. In healthy submissive dynamics, dominance is rooted in respect, consent, and the well-being of both individuals involved. Dominants are responsible for creating a safe and nurturing environment, where the submissive can explore their desires freely.

Myth 3: Submissives Lack Independence or Autonomy: Contrary to popular belief, submission does not equate to a loss of independence or autonomy. Submissives maintain their individuality, aspirations, and personal boundaries within the agreed-upon dynamics. Submissive individuals actively negotiate their limits and retain the right to voice their needs and desires, even within the submissive role.

Myth 4: Submissives Have Low Self-Worth: Another misconception is that submissives have low self-esteem or lack self-worth. On the contrary, embracing submission can be an empowering choice, allowing individuals to explore their desires, challenge societal norms, and gain a deep sense of fulfilment. Submissives often possess a strong sense of self-awareness and actively engage in personal growth.

Myth 5: Consent Is Absent in Submissive Relationships: Consent is a fundamental aspect of any healthy relationship, including submissive dynamics. It is crucial to understand that consent is an ongoing process, not a one-time agreement. Submissive individuals have the power to set boundaries, establish safe words, and withdraw consent at any time. Consent and communication form the bedrock of a responsible and respectful submissive relationship.

Myth 6: Submissives Are Always in a Submissive State: Contrary to popular belief, being a submissive does not mean that an individual is in a constant state of submission. Submissives lead multifaceted lives and engage in a variety of roles beyond their submissive identity. The submissive dynamic may be reserved for specific contexts or moments, allowing individuals to explore their desires within negotiated boundaries.

Myth 7: Submissive Relationships Lack Equality: While the power dynamics in submissive relationships may differ from traditional notions of equality, they are not inherently unequal. Consent, negotiation, and mutual respect are key elements in creating a balanced and healthy submissive dynamic. Both the submissive and dominant have responsibilities to ensure the well-being and satisfaction of all parties involved.

By dispelling common myths and stereotypes surrounding submission, we can foster a deeper understanding of the true nature of submissive relationships. Submissives are not weak or lacking agency; they are courageous individuals who actively choose to surrender control. Dominants are not inherently abusive or controlling; they are responsible for creating safe and consensual spaces. It is through debunking misconceptions that we can embrace the diversity and empowering aspects of submission, promoting healthier and more informed discussions about alternative relationship dynamics.

CHAPTER 3: THE POWER OF CHOICE: DISCUSSING THE VOLUNTARY NATURE OF SUBMISSION AND THE IMPORTANCE OF CONSENT

Submission is a voluntary and consensual choice made by individuals who seek to explore the dynamics of power exchange. In this chapter, we will delve into the power of choice within submission, emphasizing the voluntary nature of the submissive role and the vital importance of consent in establishing healthy and fulfilling relationships.

Personal Agency and Empowerment: Submission begins with personal agency and the recognition that individuals have the power to explore their desires and embrace their submissive inclinations. Choosing to be submissive is an act of empowerment, as it allows individuals to express their authentic selves and engage in relationships that align with their deepest needs and desires.

Informed Consent: Consent is the cornerstone of any healthy and ethical relationship, and it holds particular significance in submissive dynamics. It is the explicit agreement between all parties involved to willingly participate in specific activities, roles, or power dynamics. Consent is an ongoing process that requires open communication, active negotiation, and a shared understanding of boundaries and limits.

Communication and Negotiation: Open and honest communication is vital in establishing the terms and conditions of a submissive relationship. Submissives and dominants engage in thorough discussions to articulate their desires, expectations, and boundaries. Negotiation allows for the establishment of clear guidelines and ensures that all parties are actively involved in shaping the dynamics of the relationship.

Boundaries and Limits: Boundaries and limits are essential components of consent and play a crucial role in maintaining the emotional and physical well-being of all individuals involved. Submissives have the right to establish boundaries and communicate their limits to their dominant partners. It is the responsibility of the dominant to respect and honour these boundaries throughout the relationship.

Safewords and Consent Withdrawal: Safewords provide a means for submissives to communicate their needs and limits during scenes or moments of intensity. Safewords act as a signal to pause or stop activities and allow for a check-in or reassessment. Furthermore, submissives retain the right to withdraw consent at any time, and it is the responsibility of all parties to honour and respect this decision.

Continuous Consent and Aftercare: Consent is not a one-time agreement; it is an ongoing process that should be reaffirmed throughout the duration of the submissive relationship. Regular check-ins, discussions, and consent renegotiations ensure that the dynamics remain consensual and fulfilling for all individuals involved. Additionally, aftercare—a nurturing and supportive process after intense scenes—plays a vital role in addressing emotional needs and ensuring the well-being of the submissive.

Empowering Submissive Voice: Embracing the power of choice and the importance of consent empowers submissives to have an active voice in their relationships. Submissives are encouraged to express their needs, desires, and concerns openly and honestly. Their perspectives and boundaries should be valued, creating an environment that promotes trust, respect, and mutual growth.

The power of choice and the importance of consent lie at the heart of submissive relationships. Embracing submission is a voluntary and empowering decision that allows individuals to explore their desires and engage in consensual power dynamics. Through open communication, negotiation, and the establishment of boundaries, submissives and dominants create relationships built on trust, respect, and mutual growth. By honoring the power of choice and consent, we foster healthy and fulfilling submissive experiences that prioritize the well-being and agency of all parties involved.

CHAPTER 4: BUILDING TRUST: HIGHLIGHTING THE INDISPENSABLE ROLE OF TRUST IN ANY SUBMISSIVE RELATIONSHIP AND STEPS TO FOSTER IT

Trust is the cornerstone of any healthy and fulfilling submissive relationship. It forms the foundation upon which vulnerability, open communication, and the exploration of desires are built. In this chapter, we will emphasize the indispensable role of trust in submissive dynamics and explore the steps to foster and strengthen trust between submissives and dominants.

The Importance of Trust: Trust is the fundamental element that allows submissives to surrender control and embrace their vulnerability. It creates a safe space where both parties can express their desires, communicate their boundaries, and engage in power dynamics without fear of judgment or harm. Trust promotes emotional intimacy, authenticity, and the establishment of a strong connection.

Establishing Trust: Open and Honest Communication: Building trust starts with open and honest communication. Submissives and dominants should establish an environment where they feel comfortable expressing their thoughts, desires, and concerns. Active listening, non-judgmental attitudes, and empathy are key components in creating a safe space for open dialogue.

Consistency and Reliability: Consistency and reliability are crucial in building trust. Dominants must consistently demonstrate their commitment to the well-being and safety of their submissive partner.

Meeting commitments, honoring negotiated boundaries, and acting with integrity contribute to a sense of security and trustworthiness.

Transparency: Transparency involves sharing relevant information about intentions, desires, and expectations. This transparency enables submissives and dominants to make informed decisions and align their desires and boundaries effectively. Honesty and authenticity foster trust by eliminating doubts and promoting a deeper understanding of each other's needs.

Respect for Boundaries and Limits: Respecting boundaries and limits is paramount in building trust within a submissive relationship. Submissives entrust their well-being to their dominant partners, and it is essential for dominants to honour and respect the established boundaries. Clear communication and consistent adherence to negotiated limits contribute to a safe and trusting environment.

Consensual Evolution: Trust evolves through ongoing consent and communication. As the submissive dynamic progresses, desires and boundaries may evolve as well. Regular check-ins and consent renegotiations allow submissives and dominants to adapt to changing needs and ensure that trust remains intact. Embracing a consensual and adaptable approach encourages the growth and deepening of trust over time.

Vulnerability and Emotional Support: Trust flourishes when vulnerability is met with understanding and emotional support. Submissives need to feel emotionally safe to express their needs, fears, and insecurities. Dominants should provide a nurturing and supportive environment that fosters trust, empathy, and reassurance. Emotional support strengthens the bond and builds trust by creating a space where submissives can be their authentic selves.

Honouring Mistakes and Repairing Trust: Mistakes are inevitable in any relationship. When trust is breached, it is crucial to address the issue openly, take responsibility for actions, and actively work towards repairing the trust. Open communication, accountability, and a commitment to growth and learning help rebuild trust and strengthen the connection between submissives and dominants.

Time, Patience, and Consistency: Building trust takes time, patience, and consistent effort from both submissives and dominants. Trust is not established overnight but rather through a series of interactions and experiences. Patience, understanding, and a commitment to fostering trust allow for the development of a strong and resilient foundation in the submissive relationship.

Trust is the bedrock upon which submissive relationships thrive. It is established and nurtured through open communication, respect for boundaries, consistency, transparency, and emotional support.

CHAPTER 5: EFFECTIVE COMMUNICATION: EXAMINING THE SIGNIFICANCE OF OPEN DIALOGUE, NEGOTIATION, AND ESTABLISHING BOUNDARIES WITHIN THE SUBMISSIVE DYNAMIC

Effective communication is crucial in any relationship, and it holds particular significance within the context of submissive dynamics. In this chapter, we will explore the significance of open dialogue, negotiation, and the establishment of boundaries within the submissive dynamic. These practices foster understanding, consent, and a healthy exchange of desires and expectations.

Open and Honest Dialogue: Open and honest dialogue forms the foundation of effective communication within the submissive dynamic. Submissives and dominants should create a safe space where they can openly express their thoughts, desires, concerns, and emotions. This open dialogue encourages authenticity, vulnerability, and a deeper understanding of each other's needs and boundaries.

Active Listening and Empathy: Active listening is a vital aspect of effective communication. It involves fully engaging with what the other person is saying, seeking to understand their perspective, and responding empathetically. Active listening fosters a sense of validation, trust, and emotional connection. Both submissives and dominants should cultivate active listening skills to ensure that their communication is attentive and meaningful.

Negotiation and Consent: Negotiation is a collaborative process that enables submissives and dominants to define the parameters of their submissive dynamic. It involves discussing desires, expectations, boundaries, and limits, with the aim of finding mutually satisfying agreements. Negotiation allows for the establishment of consent and ensures that both parties are actively involved in shaping the dynamics of their relationship.

Establishing Clear Boundaries: Establishing clear boundaries is essential in creating a safe and consensual submissive dynamic. Boundaries serve as guidelines that define what is acceptable and what is not, both physically and emotionally. Submissives have the right to communicate their boundaries, and dominants should respect and honor them. Clear boundaries provide a sense of security, promote trust, and prevent misunderstandings or potential harm.

Non-Verbal Communication: Non-verbal communication, such as body language, gestures, and tone of voice, plays a significant role in the submissive dynamic. Submissives and dominants should be attuned to each other's non-verbal cues to better understand their partner's emotions and needs. Paying attention to non-verbal communication helps create a more nuanced and comprehensive understanding between individuals involved in the submissive relationship.

Ongoing Check-Ins: Regular check-ins are important to maintain open communication and ensure the well-being and satisfaction of all parties involved. Check-ins provide an opportunity to discuss any concerns, desires, or changes in boundaries that may have arisen. They help address potential issues early on and allow for adjustments and adaptations to be made to keep the submissive dynamic consensual and fulfilling.

Communication Tools: Safe Words and Aftercare: Safe words are a vital communication tool within the submissive dynamic. They provide submissives with a clear and concise way to communicate their needs and limits during scenes or moments of intensity. Safe words act as a signal to pause or stop activities, allowing for a check-in, adjustment, or reassessment of the situation. Aftercare, which involves nurturing and supportive actions after intense scenes, provides an opportunity for submissives to communicate their emotional needs and find comfort and reassurance.

Effective communication is the backbone of a healthy and consensual submissive relationship. Open dialogue, active listening, negotiation, and the establishment of clear boundaries foster understanding, consent, and emotional connection between submissives and dominants. Regular check-ins, non-verbal communication, and the use of communication tools such as safe words and aftercare further enhance the communication process. By prioritizing effective communication, submissives and their dominant partners can create a safe, consensual, and fulfilling dynamic that allows for the exploration of desires and the growth of their relationship.

CHAPTER 6: SAFEWORDS AND CONSENT: EXPLORING THE CRITICAL TOOLS USED TO MAINTAIN SAFETY AND WELL-BEING DURING SUBMISSIVE EXPERIENCES

Safewords and consent are critical components of maintaining safety, trust, and well-being within the context of submissive experiences. In this chapter, we will delve into the significance of safewords and consent, their role in establishing boundaries, and how they contribute to creating consensual and fulfilling submissive dynamics.

Understanding Safewords: Safewords are a vital tool used in submissive experiences to communicate boundaries, discomfort, or the need to pause or stop an activity. They provide a clear and unambiguous signal for both submissives and dominants to ensure that the dynamics remain consensual and safe. Safewords empower submissives to have agency over their experiences and allow dominants to immediately respond and adjust their actions accordingly.

Importance of Clear Communication: Clear and effective communication is essential when using safewords. Submissives should feel empowered to express themselves and use their safewords without fear of judgment or repercussions. Dominants must actively listen and respond to safewords promptly and with respect. Open dialogue before and after scenes regarding safewords ensures that both parties have a shared understanding and awareness of each other's limits and comfort levels.

Negotiating and Establishing Safewords: During the negotiation phase of a submissive dynamic, the discussion and establishment of safewords should be a priority. Submissives and dominants should collaboratively determine a safeword or a set of safewords that are easy to remember and can be clearly communicated in the heat of the moment. This negotiation process allows for the development of trust and consent, ensuring that both parties are aware of the submissives' limits and preferences.

Types of Safewords: There are different types of safewords that can be utilized depending on individual preferences and the nature of the dynamic. A common system involves using "green," "yellow," and "red" as safewords. "Green" indicates that everything is fine, "yellow" signifies a need to slow down or check in, and "red" communicates an immediate stop. Some dynamics may choose alternative words or signals to suit their needs. The key is to establish a system that is clear, understood by both parties, and enables effective communication.

Continuous Consent and Consent Withdrawal: Consent is an ongoing process throughout a submissive experience, and the use of safewords enhances this dynamic. Submissives have the right to withdraw consent at any time, even if a safeword has not been explicitly used. The withdrawal of consent may be communicated verbally or through non-verbal cues. Dominants must be attentive to the submissives' signals and promptly respond by discontinuing activities and providing support and reassurance.

Aftercare and Emotional Well-being: Safewords and consent extend beyond physical safety and encompass the emotional well-being of submissives. Aftercare, which involves nurturing and supportive actions after intense scenes, is an essential component of maintaining emotional equilibrium. It provides an opportunity for submissives to express their emotions, receive comfort, and debrief with their dominant partners. Aftercare helps foster trust, connection, and a sense of safety within the submissive dynamic.

Ongoing Communication and Adaptation: The use of safewords and consent requires ongoing communication and adaptability within the submissive dynamic. Submissives and dominants should regularly check in, discuss experiences, and explore ways to improve their communication and safety protocols. As dynamics evolve, safewords and consent may need to be reassessed and adjusted to ensure that they continue to meet the evolving needs and boundaries of all parties involved.

CHAPTER 7: SELF-DISCOVERY AND PERSONAL GROWTH: THE TRANSFORMATIVE JOURNEY OF EXPLORING SUBMISSION

The exploration of submission is a transformative journey that goes beyond the surface dynamics of power exchange. It offers individuals an opportunity for self-discovery, personal growth, and a deeper understanding of their desires, boundaries, and authentic selves. In this chapter, we will delve into the transformative aspects of exploring submission and the profound impact it can have on one's personal journey.

Embracing Authenticity: Exploring submission provides a space for individuals to embrace their authentic selves. By engaging in self-reflection and understanding their desires, needs, and boundaries, submissives can align their actions with their truest selves. Through submission, individuals can shed societal expectations and embrace their authentic desires and expressions of power exchange.

Challenging Comfort Zones: The exploration of submission often involves stepping outside of comfort zones. It requires submissives to confront fears, insecurities, and preconceived notions about power dynamics. By willingly challenging comfort zones, individuals can experience personal growth, expand their horizons, and cultivate resilience. The transformative journey of submission lies in pushing boundaries and embracing the unknown.

Self-Awareness and Emotional Intelligence: Exploring submission fosters self-awareness and emotional intelligence. Submissives develop a deeper understanding of their emotions, triggers, and responses within power dynamics. They learn to navigate and communicate their needs, desires, and boundaries effectively. This heightened self-awareness extends beyond the submissive context and can positively impact various aspects of their lives.

Communication and Emotional Expression: The exploration of submission encourages individuals to hone their communication skills and express their emotions authentically. Submissives learn to articulate their desires, boundaries, and consent effectively, while dominants practice active listening and emotional attunement. This enhanced communication and emotional expression transcend the submissive dynamic and contribute to healthier relationships in all areas of life.

Resilience and Self-Empowerment: The journey of exploring submission requires resilience and self-empowerment. Submissives learn to navigate challenges, setbacks, and emotional vulnerabilities. They discover their inner strength, develop coping mechanisms, and bounce back from adversity. Through the process of submission, individuals can reclaim agency over their desires, choices, and personal growth, ultimately empowering themselves in all aspects of life.

Embracing Vulnerability: Vulnerability is a key component of exploring submission and facilitates personal transformation. By embracing vulnerability, individuals develop a deeper connection with their own emotions, needs, and desires. They learn to trust others, cultivate intimacy, and navigate the complexities of emotional exposure. Embracing vulnerability within submission fosters personal growth and strengthens interpersonal connections.

Self-Reflection and Introspection: The transformative journey of exploring submission involves regular self-reflection and introspection. Submissives engage in introspective practices to understand their motivations, triggers, and patterns of behavior. They examine their desires, boundaries, and emotional responses, fostering personal growth, self-discovery, and a deeper understanding of themselves.

The exploration of submission is a transformative journey that extends beyond the surface-level dynamics of power exchange. Through self-discovery, personal growth, and the cultivation of authenticity, submissives embark on a profound path of self-transformation. By challenging comfort zones, enhancing self-awareness, and embracing vulnerability, individuals can navigate the complexities of submission, leading to personal empowerment, resilience, and a deeper connection with their authentic selves.

CHAPTER 8: BALANCING INDEPENDENCE AND SUBMISSION: NAVIGATING THE FINE LINE BETWEEN AUTONOMY AND RELINQUISHING CONTROL

Within the realm of submission, there exists a delicate balance between maintaining one's independence and willingly surrendering control. This chapter explores the intricacies of navigating this fine line, emphasizing the importance of autonomy, self-identity, and personal empowerment within the context of submission.

Embracing Autonomy: Autonomy is the foundation upon which a healthy and fulfilling submissive dynamic is built. It is crucial for individuals to maintain a strong sense of self, personal values, and independence while exploring submission. By embracing their autonomy, submissives can actively engage in the dynamic from a place of choice and empowerment rather than a place of surrendering their entire identity.

Defining Personal Boundaries: Establishing and communicating personal boundaries is essential for balancing independence and submission. Submissives must clearly define their limits, both physical and emotional, to ensure that their autonomy is respected. By setting boundaries, individuals assert their autonomy and create a framework within which the power exchange can occur.

Active Consent and Negotiation: Active consent and ongoing negotiation play a vital role in maintaining the balance between independence and submission. Submissives should be active participants in the negotiation process, expressing their desires, limits, and preferences. They retain the power to give or withdraw consent at any time, reaffirming their autonomy and ensuring that the dynamic aligns with their needs and boundaries.

Engaging in Self-Reflection: Self-reflection is a valuable practice for submissives to navigate the fine line between independence and submission. Regular introspection allows individuals to assess their emotions, motivations, and desires within the dynamic. By engaging in self-reflection, submissives can ensure that their engagement in submission aligns with their true selves and does not compromise their independence.

Communication and Assertiveness: Effective communication and assertiveness are essential skills for balancing independence and submission. Submissives must feel comfortable expressing their thoughts, needs, and concerns to their dominant partners. Open and honest communication helps establish a collaborative and respectful dynamic that respects both parties' autonomy and fosters a healthy power exchange.

Developing Self-Empowerment: Maintaining a sense of self-empowerment is crucial in navigating the fine line between independence and submission. Submissives should actively engage in activities and practices that promote personal growth, self-esteem, and self-care. By cultivating self-empowerment, individuals enhance their autonomy and ensure that their participation in submission is a conscious choice rather than a passive surrender.

Embracing Dynamic Evolution: Balancing independence and submission is an ongoing process that requires adaptability and flexibility. As individuals grow and evolve, their needs, desires, and boundaries may shift. It is essential for submissives to engage in regular check-ins with themselves and their dominant partners to ensure that the dynamic continues to honour their autonomy and align with their evolving sense of self.

Navigating the fine line between independence and submission is a complex and deeply personal journey. By embracing autonomy, setting clear boundaries, actively participating in consent and negotiation, engaging in self-reflection, fostering effective communication, and cultivating self-empowerment, submissives can maintain their sense of self while exploring the transformative aspects of submission. The balance between independence and submission lies in creating a dynamic that honours individual autonomy and empowers individuals to engage in submission from a place of strength and personal agency.

CHAPTER 9: RITUALS OF CONNECTION: EXPLORING THE SIGNIFICANCE OF RITUALS AND PROTOCOLS IN DEEPENING THE BOND BETWEEN DOMINANT AND SUBMISSIVE

Rituals and protocols play a significant role in deepening the bond between a dominant and a submissive. These structured practices and behaviours create a sense of connection, reinforce power dynamics, and enhance trust and intimacy within the relationship. In this chapter, we will explore the significance of rituals and protocols in the context of submission and their impact on strengthening the bond between dominants and submissives.

Understanding Rituals and Protocols: Rituals and protocols are deliberate actions, behaviours, or routines that hold symbolic meaning within the submissive dynamic. They can be physical, verbal, or symbolic in nature and are often designed to reinforce power dynamics, establish order, and enhance the connection between dominants and submissives. These practices are consensually agreed upon and can vary greatly depending on the preferences and dynamics of each relationship.

Creating a Sense of Structure and Stability: Rituals and protocols provide a sense of structure and stability within the submissive dynamic. They establish clear expectations, roles, and behaviours, allowing both dominants and submissives to navigate the relationship with a sense of purpose and direction. By incorporating rituals and protocols, the dominant-submissive bond is strengthened, and a solid foundation for trust and intimacy is built.

Reinforcing Power Dynamics: Rituals and protocols serve as a means to reinforce power dynamics within the relationship. They symbolize the roles of dominance and submission and provide a tangible expression of power exchange. For submissives, following protocols and engaging in rituals can be a way to actively submit and demonstrate their respect and devotion to their dominant partner. For dominants, enforcing protocols and witnessing submissives' adherence can reinforce their authority and sense of control.

Enhancing Trust and Intimacy: Rituals and protocols can deepen the trust and intimacy between dominants and submissives. Consistently engaging in these shared practices creates a sense of familiarity, predictability, and emotional connection. By following rituals and protocols, submissives demonstrate their trust in their dominant partner, while dominants show their commitment to fulfilling the submissives' needs and desires. These acts of mutual trust and vulnerability foster a stronger emotional bond.

Fostering Mindfulness and Presence: Rituals and protocols can encourage mindfulness and presence within the submissive dynamic. When engaging in structured actions, both dominants and submissives are encouraged to be fully present in the moment, focusing on the shared experience and the connection between them. This heightened awareness cultivates a deeper sense of intimacy and allows for a more profound connection to be forged.

Tailoring Rituals to the Relationship: Every dominant-submissive relationship is unique, and rituals and protocols should be tailored to reflect the specific dynamics and desires of the individuals involved. What holds significance and meaning for one couple may not resonate with another. It is essential for dominants and submissives to engage in open communication and negotiation to determine the rituals and protocols that enhance their connection and align with their shared vision of the relationship.

Evolving and Adapting Rituals: As the relationship grows and evolves, rituals and protocols may need to be adapted or expanded to accommodate the changing needs and dynamics of the individuals involved. Regular communication, feedback, and exploration of new rituals or adjustments to existing ones ensure that the practices continue to deepen the bond and serve the evolving connection between dominants and submissives.

Rituals and protocols serve as powerful tools for deepening the bond between dominants and submissives. They create structure, reinforce power dynamics, enhance trust and intimacy

CHAPTER 10: DAILY LIFE AS A SUBMISSIVE: POWER DYNAMICS IN EVERYDAY ROUTINES AND INTERACTIONS

The power dynamics within a dominant-submissive relationship extend far beyond intimate moments. They seep into the fabric of daily life, influencing routines, interactions, and the overall dynamics between dominants and submissives. In this chapter, we will delve into the significance of power dynamics in everyday life as a submissive, exploring how they shape routines, communication, decision-making, and the overall dynamics within the relationship.

Establishing Power Exchange in Daily Routines: Power dynamics in everyday life as a submissive often manifest through established routines. These routines can include tasks, chores, or rituals that the submissive undertakes to serve the dominant and reinforce the power exchange. By integrating power dynamics into daily routines, submissives actively participate in the dynamic and contribute to the overall balance and connection within the relationship.

Communication and Decision-Making: Power dynamics influence communication and decision-making in everyday life. Submissives may defer to their dominant partner when making decisions, seeking their guidance or approval. Clear and open communication becomes paramount as submissives express their desires, concerns, and boundaries, and dominants provide guidance and support within the established power dynamic.

Service and Submission Beyond Intimate Moments: Service and submission extend beyond intimate moments and can be incorporated into various aspects of daily life. Submissives may engage in acts of service, such as preparing meals, running errands, or organizing the household, as a way to express their submission and cater to their dominant partner's needs. These acts serve to strengthen the power dynamic and reinforce the bond between dominants and submissives.

Rituals and Protocols in Daily Life: Rituals and protocols play a significant role in daily life as a submissive. They provide structure, establish order, and enhance the power dynamics within the relationship. Submissives may engage in specific rituals or follow protocols as part of their daily routine, further deepening their submission and connection with their dominant partner.

Mindfulness and Presence: Mindfulness and presence become integral in everyday life as a submissive. Submissives are encouraged to be present in their interactions, tasks, and service to their dominant partner. By cultivating mindfulness, submissives develop a heightened awareness of their thoughts, emotions, and actions, allowing them to engage fully in their submissive role and deepen the connection with their dominant.

Negotiating Limits and Boundaries: Daily life as a submissive requires ongoing negotiation of limits and boundaries. Submissives must have open communication with their dominant partner to express their boundaries, desires, and concerns. This negotiation ensures that the power dynamics remain consensual, respectful, and aligned with the well-being and autonomy of the submissive.

Balancing Submissive Identity with Individuality: While power dynamics influence daily life, it is essential for submissives to maintain a sense of individuality and personal identity. Balancing submissive responsibilities and desires with personal needs and aspirations is crucial for the well-being and fulfilment of the submissive. Open communication, self-reflection, and regular check-ins with the dominant partner contribute to finding a harmonious balance between the submissive identity and individuality.

Power dynamics in a dominant-submissive relationship extend beyond intimate moments and permeate daily life. From established routines and communication patterns to acts of service and the integration of rituals and protocols, power dynamics shape the dynamics and interactions between dominants and submissives. Mindfulness, negotiation of boundaries, and a balanced approach to individuality within the submissive role contribute to a fulfilling and sustainable daily life as a submissive.

CHAPTER 11: REWARDS AND PUNISHMENTS: THE ROLE OF DISCIPLINE AND CONSEQUENCES IN MAINTAINING STRUCTURE AND ACCOUNTABILITY

Discipline and consequences play a crucial role in maintaining structure, accountability, and the power dynamics within a dominant-submissive relationship. In this chapter, we will explore the significance of rewards and punishments in fostering personal growth, reinforcing desired behaviours, and ensuring a healthy and consensual power exchange between dominants and submissives.

Understanding Discipline and Consequences: Discipline refers to the set of rules, expectations, and consequences that govern the submissive's behaviour within the dynamic. It provides a framework for maintaining structure, accountability, and the power dynamics between dominants and submissives. Consequences, both positive and negative, are used to reinforce or discourage specific behaviours, contributing to the overall growth and development of the submissive.

Establishing Clear Expectations: Clear expectations are crucial for effective discipline and consequences. Dominants and submissives must engage in open communication and negotiation to establish specific rules and behaviours that align with their shared vision of the dynamic. By setting clear expectations, both parties have a common understanding of the boundaries and behaviours that are expected and can be held accountable.

Positive Reinforcement: Positive reinforcement involves rewarding desired behaviours and actions. It can be in the form of praise, attention, affection, or other incentives that reinforce the submissive's positive actions. Positive reinforcement not only encourages the repetition of desirable behaviours but also fosters a sense of validation, fulfilment, and connection within the submissive dynamic.

Corrective Measures and Punishments: Corrective measures and punishments are utilized when the submissive's behaviour deviates from the established expectations or crosses defined boundaries. Punishments can take various forms, such as loss of privileges, time-outs, or other agreed-upon consequences. The purpose of punishments is not to inflict harm but to create a sense of accountability, provide an opportunity for growth, and reinforce the power dynamics within the relationship.

Consensual and Negotiated Discipline: Discipline and consequences within a dominant-submissive relationship must always be consensual and negotiated. Both dominants and submissives should have a voice in defining the rules, expectations, and consequences, ensuring that they align with their desires, boundaries, and personal growth goals. Regular check-ins, open communication, and mutual consent are crucial in maintaining a healthy and respectful disciplinary dynamic.

Promoting Personal Growth and Development: Discipline and consequences can be powerful tools for personal growth and development within the submissive dynamic. By providing structure, accountability, and opportunities for self-reflection, submissives can learn from their actions and experiences. Constructive feedback, guidance, and the reinforcement of positive behaviours contribute to the ongoing growth and evolution of the submissive.

Rebuilding Trust and Healing: Discipline and consequences can also play a role in rebuilding trust and healing within the dominant-submissive relationship. After trust has been compromised or boundaries have been crossed, carefully implemented consequences can help establish a path toward reconciliation, growth, and the restoration of trust. It is crucial for both parties to approach the process with empathy, communication, and a shared commitment to personal and relational healing.

Discipline and consequences are essential components of a healthy and consensual dominant-submissive relationship. Through clear expectations, positive reinforcement, corrective measures, and negotiated consequences, discipline provides structure, accountability, and opportunities for personal growth. It is crucial to approach discipline with respect, empathy, and open communication, ensuring that it aligns with the needs, desires, and boundaries of both dominants and submissives. When implemented responsibly, rewards and punishments can contribute to a thriving and fulfilling submissive dynamic.

CHAPTER 12: UNVEILING DESIRES: EXPLORING KINKS, FETISHES, AND BDSM PRACTICES WITH CONSENT AND NEGOTIATION

Within the realm of submission, there exists a wide array of kinks, fetishes, and BDSM practices that cater to diverse desires and fantasies. In this chapter, we will provide an overview of various practices, emphasizing the importance of consent, negotiation, and communication in exploring and engaging in these activities within a safe and consensual dominant-submissive relationship.

Understanding Kinks, Fetishes, and BDSM: Kinks, fetishes, and BDSM (Bondage, Discipline, Dominance, Submission, Sadism, Masochism) practices involve the exploration of non-traditional sexual or power dynamics. Kinks refer to unconventional sexual preferences, while fetishes involve a specific focus on objects, body parts, or activities that elicit sexual arousal. BDSM encompasses a range of activities, including bondage, impact play, role-playing, and more, where power exchange and consensual acts of dominance and submission take place.

The Importance of Consent and Negotiation: Consent and negotiation are fundamental principles in exploring kinks, fetishes, and BDSM practices. It is essential for all parties involved to give informed, enthusiastic, and ongoing consent to engage in any activity. Clear communication, negotiation of boundaries, and the establishment of safe words or signals ensure that the experiences remain consensual, respectful, and enjoyable for all participants.

Communication and Shared Desires: Open communication is key when exploring kinks, fetishes, and BDSM practices. Dominants and submissives must openly discuss their desires, boundaries, and limits to ensure that they align with their partner's expectations and comfort levels. Discussing fantasies, sharing experiences, and seeking mutual consent lay the foundation for a consensual exploration of desires and allow for a deeper connection within the dominant-submissive relationship.

Safety Precautions and Risk Awareness: Engaging in kinks, fetishes, and BDSM practices requires a thorough understanding of safety precautions and risk awareness. It is crucial to educate oneself on proper techniques, equipment usage, and potential physical and emotional risks associated with different activities. Establishing a safe environment, using consented-upon safewords or signals, and maintaining ongoing communication during play contribute to a safer and more enjoyable experience.

Aftercare and Emotional Support: Aftercare and emotional support are vital aspects of engaging in kinks, fetishes, and BDSM practices. Aftercare refers to the nurturing, comforting, and debriefing period that follows intense play or power dynamics. It includes physical and emotional care, such as cuddling, reassurance, or discussing the experience. Providing aftercare demonstrates care and respect for the well-being of the submissive and helps foster a sense of emotional connection and trust within the relationship.

Respect for Boundaries and Limits: Respecting boundaries and limits is of utmost importance in any exploration of kinks, fetishes, and BDSM practices. All parties involved must honour and adhere to the established boundaries and limits, ensuring that no one is pushed beyond their comfort zone or subjected to activities they are not willing to participate in. Regular check-ins, consent renegotiation, and ongoing communication are essential to maintaining a safe and consensual dynamic.

Continuous Learning and Growth: Exploring kinks, fetishes, and BDSM practices is an ongoing journey of learning and growth. It is essential to remain open-minded, curious, and respectful of personal boundaries and the boundaries of others. Engaging in educational resources, attending workshops or events, and seeking guidance from experienced individuals or communities can contribute to a deeper understanding and responsible exploration of desires within the submissive dynamic.

CHAPTER 13: TABOO FANTASIES AND CONSENT: NAVIGATING DARK DESIRES WITH SAFETY AND WELL-BEING

Within the realm of submission, individuals may have taboo fantasies and desires that delve into darker aspects of their sexuality. Exploring these fantasies requires careful consideration, communication, and consent to ensure the safety and well-being of all involved. In this chapter, we will address the challenges associated with taboo fantasies, emphasizing the importance of consent, negotiation, and ethical exploration within the context of a consensual dominant-submissive relationship.

Understanding Taboo Fantasies: Taboo fantasies encompass desires that are considered socially or culturally unacceptable or forbidden. These fantasies often involve elements such as role-playing, power dynamics, psychological exploration, or intense sensations. It is important to acknowledge that having taboo fantasies is a normal part of human sexuality, and exploring them within a consensual framework can be a source of personal growth and fulfilment.

Recognizing Personal Boundaries and Triggers: When exploring taboo fantasies, it is crucial to recognize and establish personal boundaries and triggers. Both dominants and submissives must engage in open and honest communication to identify any potential emotional, psychological, or physical triggers associated with the fantasies. This awareness allows for the creation of a safe and consensual space where boundaries are respected and the well-being of all participants is prioritized.

Negotiating Consent and Limits: Consent and negotiation are paramount when navigating taboo fantasies. It is essential for all parties involved to clearly communicate their desires, boundaries, and limits. Consent must be given freely and enthusiastically, and ongoing communication is necessary to ensure that boundaries are respected and that the exploration remains within the agreed-upon parameters. Regular check-ins and the use of safewords or signals provide additional layers of safety and control.

Emotional Support and Aftercare: Exploring taboo fantasies can elicit intense emotional responses and may require heightened emotional support and aftercare. Aftercare becomes even more crucial when engaging in activities that touch upon sensitive or traumatic subjects. Dominants should be attentive to the emotional well-being of their submissives, providing reassurance, comfort, and debriefing after play to facilitate emotional healing and connection.

Professional Guidance and Support: In cases where taboo fantasies involve complex psychological or traumatic themes, seeking professional guidance and support may be beneficial. Mental health professionals with expertise in alternative sexualities and BDSM can provide a safe and non-judgmental space for individuals to explore their desires, address any underlying issues, and ensure the well-being of all parties involved.

Ethical Exploration and Risk-Awareness: When engaging in taboo fantasies, it is essential to prioritize ethical exploration and risk-awareness. This involves respecting personal boundaries, ensuring informed consent, and prioritizing the emotional and physical safety of all participants. Engaging in ongoing education, understanding the potential risks and consequences, and seeking community support and resources contribute to responsible and ethical exploration.

Reflection and Self-Care: Exploring taboo fantasies can be emotionally challenging. It is crucial for all individuals involved to engage in self-reflection and self-care throughout the process. This may involve setting aside time for self-reflection, practicing self-compassion, seeking support from trusted individuals or communities, and prioritizing personal well-being outside of the submissive dynamic.

Exploring taboo fantasies within a consensual dominant-submissive relationship requires careful attention to consent, negotiation, and ethical exploration. By acknowledging personal boundaries and triggers, engaging in open communication, seeking professional guidance when necessary, and prioritizing emotional support and aftercare, individuals can navigate the challenges of exploring darker desires while ensuring the safety and well-being of all involved. Responsible and consensual exploration can lead to personal growth, healing, and the deepening of the submissive dynamic.

CHAPTER 14: NAVIGATING LIMITS: UNDERSTANDING HARD AND SOFT LIMITS IN THE SUBMISSIVE CONTEXT

In any submissive dynamic, it is crucial to recognize and respect personal limits. Limits refer to the boundaries and restrictions that individuals have in terms of their comfort, physical well-being, emotional safety, and psychological boundaries. In this chapter, we will delve into the significance of hard and soft limits within the submissive context and explore strategies for effectively managing and navigating them.

Understanding Hard Limits: Hard limits are the absolute boundaries that a submissive is unwilling or unable to cross. They are non-negotiable and must be respected at all times. Hard limits can vary greatly from person to person and may involve specific activities, triggers, or experiences that individuals simply cannot or do not wish to engage in. It is crucial for both dominants and submissives to clearly communicate and acknowledge each other's hard limits.

Identifying Soft Limits: Soft limits, in contrast to hard limits, are boundaries that a submissive may be willing to explore under certain circumstances or with further negotiation and consent. They are areas where individuals may have reservations or concerns but are open to discussion and potential expansion. Identifying and discussing soft limits provide an opportunity for growth and exploration within the submissive dynamic while maintaining a sense of safety and consent.

Communicating Limits Effectively: Effective communication is key when it comes to navigating limits within a submissive context.

Submissives should feel empowered to express their limits openly and honestly, while dominants should create a safe and non-judgmental space for open dialogue. Both parties should actively listen and validate each other's boundaries, ensuring that the submissive's limits are respected and considered in all aspects of the dynamic.

Negotiation and Consent: Negotiation and consent are crucial components of managing limits within the submissive dynamic. When exploring soft limits, it is important for both dominants and submissives to engage in ongoing negotiation, discussing the potential scenarios, boundaries, and precautions associated with the desired activities. Consent must be enthusiastic, informed, and continuously given, ensuring that both parties have a clear understanding of each other's limits and desires.

Regular Check-Ins and Consent Renegotiation: Limits may evolve and change over time, and it is essential to engage in regular check-ins and consent renegotiation within the submissive dynamic. As individuals grow and develop within their roles, it is important to reassess boundaries, explore new desires, and communicate any shifts in comfort levels. Regular communication and check-ins contribute to maintaining a healthy, consensual, and evolving submissive dynamic.

Utilizing Safewords and Signals: Safewords and signals are invaluable tools for managing limits and ensuring the safety and well-being of all participants. Submissives should have a clear and agreed-upon safeword or signal that allows them to communicate their boundaries or the need to pause or stop an activity. Dominants should be attentive and responsive to the use of safewords or signals, ensuring immediate cessation of the activity and providing care and support to the submissive.

Trust and Emotional Support: Building and maintaining trust is paramount when navigating limits within the submissive dynamic. Submissives should feel secure in expressing their boundaries, knowing that their limits will be respected. Dominants should provide emotional support and reassurance, creating an environment where submissives feel safe and empowered to communicate their limits openly. Trust and emotional support foster a healthy and consensual exploration of limits within the submissive context.

Navigating limits within the submissive context requires open communication, negotiation, and consent. By understanding and respecting hard and soft limits, engaging in ongoing check-ins and consent renegotiation, utilizing safewords or signals, and fostering a foundation of trust and emotional support, individuals can effectively manage and navigate their boundaries within the submissive dynamic. By doing so, they can create a safe, consensual, and fulfilling submissive experience for all involved parties.

CHAPTER 15: SUBMISSION AND PERSONAL EMPOWERMENT: THE TRANSFORMATIVE EFFECTS BEYOND SEXUAL ENCOUNTERS

While submission is often associated with sexual dynamics, embracing submission can have transformative effects that extend beyond the realm of sexual encounters. In this chapter, we will explore the empowering aspects of submission and discuss how it can positively impact personal growth, self-awareness, and overall well-being.

Redefining Power and Strength: Contrary to societal norms, submission challenges the traditional notions of power and strength. It emphasizes that true strength lies in vulnerability, trust, and the ability to surrender control. By embracing submission, individuals redefine their understanding of power, recognizing that it can be found in letting go and allowing another person to guide and support them.

Developing Self-Awareness: Submission provides a unique opportunity for individuals to explore their desires, boundaries, and emotions on a deep level. By surrendering control, submissives gain insights into their own needs, fears, and motivations. This heightened self-awareness allows them to make informed choices, set clearer boundaries, and navigate their personal journey with a deeper understanding of themselves.

Building Trust and Intimacy: Submission fosters an environment of trust and intimacy within the dominant-submissive relationship. By entrusting their well-being and desires to their dominant partner, submissives create a foundation of trust that extends beyond sexual encounters. This trust cultivates emotional closeness, open communication, and a profound sense of connection, enhancing the overall quality of the relationship.

Emotional Healing and Growth: Submission can provide a healing and growth-oriented space for individuals who have experienced trauma or emotional challenges. By engaging in consensual power dynamics, submissives can reclaim control over their own experiences and rewrite their narratives. The support, understanding, and care received from their dominant partner can facilitate emotional healing and foster personal growth.

Increased Self-Confidence: Embracing submission can boost self-confidence by allowing individuals to explore and express their desires authentically. The affirmation and validation received from their dominant partner contribute to a positive self-image and a stronger sense of self-worth. As submissives gain confidence in their ability to communicate their needs and embrace their desires, their overall self-confidence and self-assuredness grow.

Empowerment through Choice: Contrary to popular misconceptions, submission is a choice. Submissives have the power to set their own boundaries, negotiate consent, and explore activities that align with their desires and comfort levels. By actively engaging in the decision-making process, submissives reclaim their agency and experience a profound sense of empowerment.

Integrating Submission into Daily Life: The transformative effects of submission can extend into daily life beyond intimate moments. Submissives can incorporate elements of submission, such as mindfulness, service, and respect, into their routines and interactions. This integration allows them to embody the principles of submission, leading to personal growth, enhanced relationships, and a greater sense of purpose and fulfilment.

Embracing submission can have profound effects that go beyond sexual encounters. By redefining power, fostering self-awareness, building trust and intimacy, facilitating emotional healing and growth, boosting self-confidence, empowering through choice, and integrating submission into daily life, individuals can experience personal empowerment and transformative growth. Submission becomes a powerful tool for self-discovery, personal development, and overall well-being.

CHAPTER 16: SUBMISSIVE PARTNERSHIPS: DYNAMICS, BENEFITS, AND CHALLENGES OF LONG-TERM RELATIONSHIPS

Long-term submissive relationships involve a deep commitment between a dominant and a submissive, where the power dynamic extends beyond individual encounters and becomes an integral part of their partnership. In this chapter, we will explore the dynamics, benefits, and challenges of long-term submissive relationships, shedding light on the unique experiences and considerations that arise within these partnerships.

Establishing a Strong Foundation: Building a strong foundation is crucial for the success of any long-term submissive relationship. This involves open and honest communication, shared values and goals, mutual respect, and a deep understanding of each other's needs and desires. Establishing a solid foundation creates a framework for trust, growth, and the ongoing development of the submissive dynamic.

Deepening Trust and Intimacy: Long-term submissive relationships provide the opportunity to deepen trust and intimacy over time. As the relationship progresses, the dominant and submissive gain a profound understanding of each other's vulnerabilities, desires, and boundaries. This deepened trust allows for a heightened level of emotional and physical intimacy, creating a strong bond between partners.

Growth and Personal Development: Long-term submissive relationships offer a fertile ground for personal growth and development. The ongoing exploration of desires, limits, and dynamics provides opportunities for self-discovery, self-improvement, and self-actualization. Both the dominant and submissive can learn and evolve together, supporting each other's journeys of personal growth and transformation.

Stability and Consistency: Long-term submissive relationships often provide a sense of stability and consistency that can be comforting and fulfilling for both partners. The established roles, rituals, and protocols create a structure within which the power dynamic operates, fostering a sense of security and predictability. This stability allows for the deepening of trust and the exploration of more profound submissive experiences.

Emotional Support and Connection: In long-term submissive relationships, emotional support and connection are vital. The dominant partner provides guidance, care, and understanding to the submissive, creating a safe space for vulnerability and emotional expression. The connection between partners deepens as they navigate challenges, share experiences, and support each other's emotional well-being.

Challenges of Long-Term Commitment: Long-term submissive relationships are not without challenges. The power dynamics can occasionally create tensions or misunderstandings that require open communication and negotiation to address. Maintaining a healthy balance between autonomy and submission can also be challenging, as both partners continue to grow and evolve individually. Ongoing effort and commitment are necessary to navigate these challenges effectively.

Evolving Desires and Compatibility: As time passes, desires and interests may evolve for both the dominant and submissive partners. It is crucial for partners to engage in ongoing communication and renegotiation to ensure their desires and compatibility remain aligned. Flexibility, understanding, and a willingness to adapt to changing needs contribute to the longevity and satisfaction of the submissive partnership.

Long-term submissive relationships offer a unique and profound connection between partners. With a strong foundation, deepened trust and intimacy, opportunities for growth and personal development, stability and consistency, emotional support and connection, as well as the ability to navigate challenges and evolving desires, these partnerships can provide a fulfilling and transformative experience for both the dominant and submissive.

CHAPTER 17: COMMUNITY AND SUPPORT: NURTURING GROWTH AND UNDERSTANDING IN THE SUBMISSIVE JOURNEY

Finding a supportive community and accessing resources are essential aspects of the submissive journey. In this chapter, we will explore the importance of community and support in fostering personal growth, providing understanding, and navigating the challenges and triumphs of a submissive lifestyle.

The Power of Community: Being part of a supportive community of like-minded individuals can be incredibly empowering for submissives. A community provides a safe space for sharing experiences, seeking advice, and receiving validation. It allows submissives to connect with others who understand their desires, challenges, and triumphs, creating a sense of belonging and camaraderie.

Resources for Education and Understanding: Accessing resources such as books, websites, workshops, and educational events is vital for deepening understanding and expanding knowledge within the submissive journey. These resources offer valuable information on various aspects of submission, including communication, negotiation, safety, and exploring different dynamics and practices. They provide submissives with the tools they need to navigate their journey with awareness and confidence.

Online Communities and Forums: Online communities and forums provide a platform for submissives to connect with others from around the world, regardless of geographical location. These platforms offer opportunities for discussion, sharing experiences, and seeking advice in a supportive and anonymous environment. Engaging in online communities allows submissives to learn from diverse perspectives, broaden their horizons, and gain insights from individuals with varying levels of experience.

Local Support Groups and Events: Seeking out local support groups and attending events can be a valuable way to connect with individuals within the submissive community on a more personal level. These groups and events offer opportunities for in-person interaction, discussions, workshops, and socializing. Engaging with local support groups allows submissives to build lasting connections, exchange knowledge, and receive direct support within their own communities.

Mentoring and Guidance: Finding a mentor or a trusted guide within the submissive community can provide invaluable support and guidance. Mentors, with their experience and wisdom, can offer insights, advice, and personalized assistance to submissives, helping them navigate challenges, clarify goals, and embrace their submissive journey with confidence. Mentoring relationships foster personal growth, self-reflection, and the sharing of knowledge within the submissive community.

Professional Support: In some cases, seeking professional support, such as therapy or counselling, can be beneficial for submissives. Professional therapists who specialize in relationships, sexuality, or BDSM can provide a non-judgmental and supportive space for submissives to explore their desires, process challenges, and address any emotional or psychological concerns that may arise within their submissive journey.

Developing a Supportive Network: Building a supportive network of friends, partners, and confidants within the submissive community is crucial for ongoing support and growth. These individuals understand the dynamics and challenges of the submissive lifestyle and can provide guidance, empathy, and encouragement. Nurturing these relationships fosters a sense of belonging, mutual support, and personal growth within the submissive journey.

Finding a supportive community and accessing resources are essential components of the submissive journey. Engaging with a community provides a sense of belonging, understanding, and validation. Utilizing educational resources, online communities, local support groups, mentoring relationships, professional support, and building a supportive network contribute to personal growth, self-awareness, and the ability to navigate the challenges and triumphs of the submissive lifestyle. Remember, you are not alone in your journey, and support is available to help you thrive and embrace your submissive identity

EPILOGUE: A CONTINUATION OF THE JOURNEY

As we come to the end of our exploration in "Unveiling Submission: Embracing the Power of Surrender," we find ourselves at the crossroads of reflection and anticipation. The pages before us have been filled with insights, revelations, and moments of profound connection. We have delved into the depths of submission, unearthing its intricacies, and embracing its transformative power.

But this is not the end of the journey; rather, it is a continuation—a stepping stone to further growth, understanding, and self-discovery. The path of submission is an ever-evolving one, shaped by individual experiences, relationships, and personal desires.

As you close this book, remember that the exploration of submission is a deeply personal endeavour. Your journey will be unique, moulded by your own desires, boundaries, and experiences. Embrace the power of choice, the strength of open communication, and the importance of consent in all aspects of your journey.

Seek out like-minded individuals, supportive communities, and resources that nourish your growth and understanding. Surround yourself with those who embrace the beauty of submission and respect your authentic self. Remember that vulnerability is not a weakness but a source of empowerment, and that through surrender, you can discover hidden depths within yourself.

As you navigate the complexities of power dynamics, continue to nurture trust, communicate openly, and establish clear boundaries. Regularly check in with yourself and your partner(s), ensuring that the path you tread remains one of mutual satisfaction, growth, and fulfilment.

Know that your desires, fantasies, and kinks are valid, and that consent and negotiation are the guiding stars of your journey. Embrace the taboo and explore the edges of darkness, but always prioritize the safety and well-being of yourself and those you engage with.

Above all, never forget that submission extends beyond the bedroom—it is a way of being, a mindset that influences every facet of your life. Embrace the lessons learned, the transformations experienced, and the deep connections forged, as you navigate the balance between independence and surrender.

So, as you step forward into the continuation of your journey, carry with you the wisdom gleaned from these pages. Embrace the power of surrender, the beauty of vulnerability, and the authenticity of your desires. May your path be one of self-discovery, growth, and connection, as you continue to unveil the depths of your own submission.

Remember that the power lies within you, waiting to be embraced and celebrated. May you find fulfilment, liberation, and profound connection as you continue to navigate the intricate dance of dominance and submission.

Farewell for now, but know that this is not the end. The journey of unveiling submission is ongoing—a tapestry of exploration that knows no bounds. Embrace it, embrace yourself, and continue to write your own story—one that embraces the power of surrender and the vast possibilities that lie within.

Until we meet again on the next chapter of your journey, may the power of submission guide you, inspire you, and lead you towards the fulfilment you seek.

Bella x

57